Surrogacy

An Essential Guide to the Surrogacy Process, Surrogacy Costs, and Finding a Surrogate Mother

by Dianne Whitfield

Table of Contents

Introduction

Surrogacy can be a viable option for couples who, for some reason, cannot go through the process of pregnancy or delivering a child. Surrogacy has been a controversial topic worldwide because of its social, moral, and personal implications. What are the valid reasons that can defend a couple's right to surrogacy? When can couples resort to surrogacy? Are you qualified to choose surrogacy as an option of nurturing a family? These are only few of the vital questions that you need to answer. To answer these, and to decide if surrogacy is for you, you have to understand what surrogacy is all about.

Some couples have chosen the path to surrogacy without fully knowing the pros and cons of it, and were assailed by unexpected problems afterwards. There are times that couples are not prepared for the added responsibility, and they simply crumble amidst the seemingly Herculean task.

This book can provide all the essential information you need if you're considering surrogacy for your family. You will learn how to go about surrogacy and what to expect in the process, including the costs and possible complications.

Chapter 1: Understanding Surrogacy

Choosing surrogacy to experience the joys of parenthood is just one option for couples who are unable to conceive or bear children naturally. Couples diagnosed with infertility, or those who potentially risk their health with pregnancy, are now more likely to consider surrogacy over adoption.

What is surrogacy?

Surrogacy is the process where a pre-selected woman agrees to carry and deliver a baby for another couple, who will then nurture and raise the baby as their own.

Types of Surrogacy According to Method

Gestational surrogacy – In gestational surrogacy, the surrogate mother is not biologically related to the child. The child is typically conceived from the egg of the intended mother and the sperm of the intended father. A donor egg or sperm is sometimes used when one of the intended parents is unable to provide one.

Through in-vitro fertilization (IVF), the ovum and sperm of the biological parents are combined and fertilized in a laboratory for at least three days. Afterwards, the embryo is implanted in the surrogate mother's womb so that the baby can be nurtured to full-term until delivered successfully.

With gestational surrogacy, the intended (or one of the intended) parents are also the child's biological parents. As the surrogate mother is not biologically related to the child she is carrying, she has less of an emotional attachment to the child. This lessens the possibility of complications down the road.

Traditional surrogacy – In this type of surrogacy, the surrogate mother is the biological mother of the child. Her egg or ovum is fertilized with sperm from the intended father or an anonymous donor through artificial insemination.

Traditional surrogacy is comparatively easier and less costly since the process of in-vitro fertilization for gestational surrogacy is more complex.

Types of Surrogacy According to Purpose

1. **Altruistic** – In this type of surrogacy, the surrogate agrees not to receive compensation for carrying the child. No payment is expected because it is understood that the primary purpose is to help others, typically a childless couple, enlarge their family. Nonetheless, the parties involved agree that all expenses incurred during the pregnancy and delivery will be paid by the intended parents or parents-to-be. This type is of surrogacy is approved in many countries and in many states in the US.

2. **Commercial** – With commercial surrogacy, a woman agrees to be a surrogate mother in exchange for monetary compensation. Acting as a surrogate in order to generate income is primarily banned in all states in the US, and is considered illegal by almost all countries in the world. The law contends that surrogacy should be done for humane reasons and not for the purpose of making big money.

Reasons Why Couples Choose Surrogacy:

> ➤ The intended mother has a medical condition or illness in which pregnancy is contraindicated. She is most likely unable

to carry the baby to term or deliver the baby normally because of an illness. Some examples of these illnesses are increased risks of spontaneous abortion, cardiovascular conditions, and pulmonary hypertension.

➢ The woman doesn't want to undergo the pains of carrying the baby to full-term and/or delivery.

➢ The woman is unable to conceive due to unknown reasons, although she has not been diagnosed with a reproductive dysfunction.

➢ The woman has a career that makes pregnancy impossible.

➢ LGBT couples who are of the same sex.

➢ When the woman is under medication that is contraindicated in pregnancy.

➢ Couples who are past reproductive age.

➤ Recurrent pregnancy loss and spontaneous abortion.

➤ A dysfunction in the womb of the female such as those who had undergone hysterectomy (removal of the uterus).

➤ Failure of in-vitro implantations.

➤ Infertility of either one or both partners.

These are only a few of the reasons why others have chosen surrogacy. Typically, these are also among the reasons that prompt some couples to consider adoption. The most compelling reasons for couples to decide to go for surrogacy versus adoption are (1) the child will likely have a biological relationship with the intended parents and (2) the intended parents can monitor the health and growth of both the baby and the surrogate mother.

Chapter 2: Guidelines to the Surrogacy Process

Surrogacy guidelines vary for each US state and for each country. In the US, some states fully support surrogacy with legitimate companies being responsible with matching surrogate mothers to couples. Not all states do, though. Some do not support the legislation for surrogacy so you'll have to check your own county's rules. However, there are general guidelines that you should know when deciding to go into surrogacy.

<ins>General Guidelines to the Surrogacy Process:</ins>

1. **Everyone concerned should give their express, informed consent.**

   In the event of unforeseen complications, you will want to have a legal and binding contract that has all the details of your surrogacy agreement. Seek the help of a lawyer to prepare a binding contract of agreement.

   The contract or agreement must signify the voluntary and express informed consent of all the signatories. The signatories should include the intended parents, the surrogate mother, the donors and doctors involved if possible, and legal witnesses. Care must be made to ensure everyone understands every sentence included in the contract and that everyone is signing voluntarily.

Ensure that all legal documents are in order before starting the process.

2. **Understand your rights to surrogacy in accordance with federal and state laws.**
In the US constitution, surrogacy falls under the fifth and the fourteenth amendments. The Fifth Amendment covers the right to privacy, including the freedom to procreate and the right to raise children the way the parents deem fit. The right to hire a surrogate mother is also included in the fifth. The 14th Amendment concerns Equal Protection rights, but there are certain states that don't support this right when it comes to surrogacy.

Since the laws about surrogacy vary from state to state, consult a lawyer who can legalize your surrogacy to ensure that every step you do is protected by law.

As of this writing, bans on surrogacy are enforced in the US states of Arizona and the District of Columbia. States that allow but regulate surrogacy are: Arkansas, Florida, Illinois, Nevada, New Hampshire, Texas, Utah, and Virginia. States considered surrogate-friendly are Maryland and California. The rest of the states didn't ban surrogacy but they sometimes void, penalize, and are inconsistent about their support.

For complete details on the law of each US state regarding surrogacy, visit these websites:

http://www.thesurrogacyexperience.com/surrogate-mothers/the-law/u-s-surrogacy-law-by-state/

https://www.americanprogress.org/issues/women/news/2007/12/17/3758/guide-to-state-surrogacy-laws/

3. **Observe the age requirements**

The age bracket for surrogate mothers is from 21 years old to 40 years old. Of course, she must be healthy mentally, physically, and emotionally. She must also have at least one biological child. It goes without saying that you have to personally choose your child's surrogate mother to ensure that your baby will be healthy and safe. The qualifications of the surrogate mother are discussed in detail in Chapter 4.

nsult with licensed counselors

rogacy guidelines require the couple and the
ogate mother to undergo counseling before and
after the surrogacy process.

5. **The surrogate mother is required to attend support groups**

This is another necessary guideline that is included to ensure that the surrogate mother will be ready for the surrogacy process. Spending time with a support group will allow the surrogate mother to feel that the process is not something to be afraid of. You and your partner as the intended parents may also attend if you feel the need to.

6. **Complete the necessary medical and psychological screening procedures**

This guideline is important especially in selecting the biological parents of the baby and in the selection of the surrogate mother. The needed tests are specified in Chapter 4.

Chapter 3: Surrogacy Costs

Surrogacy costs vary depending on the type of surrogacy you decide on. Choosing a relative from the intended mother's side of the family as a surrogate mother using the traditional method of artificial insemination can reduce the cost. It's also generally more convenient for all parties concerned.

How much does surrogacy cost?

How much you will need to spend is undoubtedly one of your top considerations as a couple opting for surrogacy. The costs will differ based on the following:

> ➤ **Surrogacy Agencies** – Agencies cost from around $70,000 to $150,000 depending on the type of surrogacy that you choose. The cost may be inclusive of all insurances, medical, attorney and surrogate fees.

If you do not plan on going through an agency, here is a list of things you need to prepare for and the estimated costs:

> ➤ **Transfer of embryo** = $1,000

- ➤ **Pre-natal care** = $2,000 to $3,000 (without health insurance)

- ➤ **Normal hospital delivery expenses** = $10,000 (exclusive of other services) and around $30,000 (inclusive of hospital care)

- ➤ **Living expenses** = $30,000 to $45,000 ($3,000 per month after confirmation of baby's heartbeat up to delivery)

- ➤ **Mandatory Support Group meetings** = $1,200 ($100 per month)

- ➤ **Miscellaneous expenses** = $2,000 to $2,400 ($200 per month)

- ➤ **Attorney's fees** = $4,000 to $5,000

- ➤ **Insurance fees** = $30,000 to $40,000 (This is largely dependent on the type of insurance you want the surrogate mother to have. It can include life insurance for your benefit and that of her family in case the surrogate mother dies.)

➢ **Maternity clothing allowance** = $1,000 to $1,500 (You can increase or decrease this expenditure based on your own judgment.)

➢ **Psychological screening and background check** = $1,250 to $1,500 (You need this to ensure that your surrogate mother is of sound mind and has no criminal records.)

➢ **Cesarean operation fee** = $50,000 to $60,000 (Be ready with this amount of money if your surrogate mother has to undergo a cesarean section operation to deliver your baby. Medical insurance will lessen the amount you pay to around $20,000 to $30,000.)

These are the usual fees incurred in traditional surrogacy. Gestational surrogacy is a little more expensive. There may be additional fees in other states that are not included. You will have to consider adding exigency budgets. These fees don't include the baby's care after the delivery. These are also subject to inflation.

Chapter 4: Finding a Surrogate Mother

Finding a surrogate mother is the most crucial step in the surrogacy process. You can go through agencies or do it independently. Here are some guidelines you can follow.

1. **Consider relatives or friends as a surrogate mother**

     This can be your first option for traditional surrogacy, if you're confident that there will be no ensuing problems. This will be less expensive than going to a surrogate agency or finding a surrogate mother yourself.

     If the surrogate mother is a relative of the man, ensure that they are only related by marriage and not by blood. This is done in consideration of the scientific fact that the combination of genes between close relatives can cause abnormalities in the offspring. For this reason, siblings and relatives of the man up to the second degree of consanguinity should not be considered as surrogate mothers no matter how normal they are. The detrimental effects will be evident only once the genes combine with one another.

If you have chosen gestational surrogacy, you still have to be cautious not to pair closely related ovum and sperm cells because of the danger of eventual abnormalities in the baby.

2. Use an agency to find a surrogate mother

The agency acts as the middle man in connecting you to a qualified and appropriate surrogate mother. The agency does all the screening of the candidates, and you'll have to pay the agency for its services and that of the surrogate mother. This is convenient for couples who don't want to be bothered with the details of the process. It's more expensive, though, because you're going through a third party.

3. Find your baby's ideal surrogate mother independently

You can find a surrogate mother for your baby on your own. If you're doing the selection of the surrogate mother, these are things that you must consider:

Aspects to consider when choosing a sur. mother

> **Age** – She must be at least 21 years old and not older than 40 years old. Some surrogacy clinics accept older or younger women, but they're still screened comprehensively. It's advisable, though, that when you choose independently you should stick to the age requirement. Too young or too old surrogate mothers usually increase the risk of the baby developing future health problems.

> **Health** - She must be healthy physically, mentally, and emotionally. In addition to passing the usual physical and medical diagnostic tests, take note that she also has to be tested negative for diseases that can be inherited such as HIV and syphilis. Likewise, she has to pass the psychological test conducted by a licensed mental expert to ascertain that she's emotionally and mentally stable.

She must undergo immunity for measles, chicken pox, and other neonatal-prone diseases.

valuation of her reproductive organs
ust be done to determine if she's
capable of carrying a baby to full-term and
if she can deliver the baby with minimal
risks. One necessary requirement is that
she must have already delivered a healthy
baby—without any complications—at
least once.

➤ **Voluntary participation** – She has given
informed consent and has voluntarily
participated after learning all about her
responsibilities as a surrogate mother. She
must also know the risks of pregnancy
and birthing and the fact that she has to
give all her rights once the baby has been
successfully delivered. She must be aware
of all the responsibilities of being a
surrogate mother.

➤ **Stable lifestyle** – She may not live
affluently, but she should at least have a
stable lifestyle and a sound economic
condition.

➤ **Weight** – Her weight must be ideal for
her height. You can refer to the BMI
(Body-Mass Index) chart to determine
this. She must not be overweight or

underweight. Generally, her
not be lower than 100 pou
height is 5 feet, her weighı
between 100 pounds to 120 ¡
her height is 5'4", her weight   ᴗᴄ
within 110 pounds to 140 pounds. If her
height is 5'6", her weight must be from
120 to 150 pounds.

➢ **No vices** – She must not be addicted to
any drug or medication. She must not be a
smoker or an alcoholic and must not be
on any illegal drugs.

➢ **No criminal records** – The surrogate,
and if possible, her immediate family,
must have a spotless record with no
history of violence or social
misdemeanors.

➢ **Intelligence Quotient (IQ)** – Of course,
you would want your baby to be
intelligent. Choose a woman with an
above average IQ, or at least an average
IQ.

➤ **Physical traits** – It's natural that parents want their children to look good. Choosing a beautiful surrogate mother is not a sin. Remember that physical traits are also inherited.

On the other hand, the character of the surrogate mother must always take precedence over her physical appearance. She may be a striking beauty but if her character is questionable, then you may want to find other candidates.

➤ **Family history** – You have to determine too if there are any family histories of medical and mental conditions that are not apparent in the surrogate mother but can be passed on to her offspring. Be judicious in going over the surrogate mother's family history.

4. **Prepare a contract**

Whether you're going through an agency, through your relatives and friends, or choosing the surrogate mother on your own, you'll have to prepare a surrogacy contract that will protect your rights, the rights of the surrogate, and that of the child's. Th[...] also to prevent subsequent legal issues.

Again, since state laws differ, you have to double check that all items are covered in the surrogacy contract. Some states require that the intended parents adopt the baby from the surrogate mother, while other states allow the declaration of parentage of the intended parents as soon as the baby is born.

The items that should be included in the contract are the following:

> **Obligations or responsibilities of the surrogate mother.** This must be clearly stated and specified.

> **Obligations or responsibilities of the future parents**. This must also be specified item by item.

> **Financial agreement.** A detailed and itemized financial allotment that will show what the intended parents must pay and what the surrogate mother will get in return. The cost must be in numerical figures and can be computed. Excessive

es are prohibited in most US states and other countries.

> **Alternative actions in case of unexpected occurrences** such as the birth of twins or triplets, death of the baby, death of the mother, refusal of the surrogate mother to part with the baby, complete abandonment of the baby by the surrogate mother to the intended parents, and similar events.

> **Agreement after delivery**. Indicate what is expected from the surrogate mother after delivering the baby. Will there be visitation rights, or should the mother cut all ties with the baby after delivery? All terms should be stated clearly in the contract.

Hire a competent lawyer who is well-versed with the surrogacy process in your particular state, so that all areas that have to be covered are included in your contract. In this aspect, hiring a lawyer is a must.

Chapter 5: Necessary Steps to Take

The traits that make an ideal surrogate mother are presented in Chapter 4. Agencies will do most of the monitoring if you decide to make use of one. Your responsibility is to pay the required fees for each of the steps. If you have decided to manage the traditional surrogacy process independently, here is a summary of the steps that you have to accomplish.

Step #1 – Know the specific guidelines in your state or country

There is no federal law involving surrogacy in the US. If you live outside of the US, you can visit your government agencies to learn about these surrogacy guidelines. Each country has its own guidelines on surrogacy. India and Russia supports surrogacy, while Australia and Canada allows altruistic surrogacy. In Iceland and Italy, all forms of surrogacy are illegal.

Step #2 - Discuss and plan your choices with your partner

You and your partner have to agree on all your decisions 100%. Will you go through an agency, select from a relative or friend, or will you do the screening of the surrogate

es? These are among the things you must
.e agreement on before you can proceed.

.p #3 – Draw up a profile of your ideal surrogate mother

Decide what traits you want in a surrogate mother. Do you have any preferences and requirements? Understandably, good mental and physical health should be number one on your list. What about the physical aspects? What traits do you prefer? How many children should the mother have had first? Create a checklist with the non-negotiables clearly identified along with traits that you desire but can give wiggle room for. This will facilitate your selection and help you decide your top candidates.

Step #4 – Meet the prospective surrogate mothers

After determining what to look for, you should arrange a meeting with the prospective surrogate mothers. Interview them to get a glimpse of their personalities from your conversations. You can get an inkling of their thoughts from their answers to your queries. Ask them how they feel about the whole surrogacy process. Look into the surrogate mothers' eligibility (age, had at least one child, and other qualifications mentioned in Chapter 4.)

Step #5 – Conduct a complete assessment of the surrogate mother

Select three candidates from the potential surrogate mothers based on your initial assessment. Conduct a more intensive interview and character assessment. Get to really know them personally and if possible, ask a medical practitioner to start physical, medical, mental, and personality assessments with all three of them. For gestational surrogacy, the egg cells must be acquired from the donor at this point.

Step #6 – Conduct a medical check-up for the sperm donor (father-to-be)

If you haven't done this yet, then the husband or sperm donor has to undergo a medical assessment to determine if his sperm is healthy and strong enough to survive artificial insemination or in-vitro fertilization.

In gestational surrogacy, the male and female counterparts must undergo the same assessment to determine if they're both qualified to donate eggs and sperms as biological parents for the in-vitro fertilization. The surrogate mother must also be ready to carry the fertilized egg in her womb.

Step #7 - Draw a contract through a lawyer

Once the chosen woman is fit to become a surrogate mother, a contract must be drawn through a lawyer to specify the responsibilities of both parties. The contract has to specify each of the responsibilities of the surrogate mother and the intended parents.

Step #8 – Schedule the procedure with your doctor

Your doctor will set the most optimal dates to perform artificial insemination (for traditional surrogacy) or in-vitro fertilization (for gestational surrogacy).

Step #9 - Monitor the pregnancy of the surrogate mother

When the fertilization process is complete, start monitoring the progress of the surrogate's pregnancy. Join her in her visits to the obstetrician regularly to ensure that the baby's development and growth are normal. The doctor usually prescribes multivitamins and food supplements for the pregnant mother. Be sure your financial obligations include all these until the term of the baby has been completed.

Step #10 – Prepare for the baby's arrival

Know when the expected delivery day is and be there. If this is not possible, then you can monitor the situation through constant contact with her doctor or medical worker.

Step #11 – Complete contractual or state requirements

In some states, it's required for the intended parents to adopt the baby from the surrogate mother, and the adoption can only be possible after the mandatory waiting period.

You will typically go through fewer steps if you choose to work with an agency, because most of them will be done by the agency in your behalf. All you have to do is to file your application, provide necessary documents, pay, and then sign a contract. Before you do that though, ask an attorney to go over the contract with you. Iron out chinks with the agency before signing the contract.

Chapter 6: Important Pointers on Surrogacy

This list will further help you anticipate and prepare for possible complications in surrogacy. By being mindfully aware and prepared for anything, you can be among the many *many* couples who are now enjoying family life with their children through surrogacy:

1. **Numerous lawsuits have stemmed from surrogacy**. There are, by far, more successful surrogacies than not, but it helps to be aware of the fact that some do end in lawsuits. This is so you will prepare your contract judiciously. Check and double check with your lawyer to make sure you don't leave any loopholes that can get you sued.

2. **Be aware of the health risks to your baby**. It's imperative that you perform medical and psychiatric screening thoroughly on the potential surrogate mothers before finally choosing one. The same is true with the sperm donor. Whether the sperm is donated by the father-to-be or an anonymous donor, you must be aware that the sperm has the potential to cause health issues that might not be detected until after the baby is born.

3. **Ensure that the contract protects all parties concerned.** Your interests and that of the mother must not be affected negatively. The surrogate mother can be considered a family member while the surrogacy process is ongoing and must be treated fairly and justly.

4. **Choose agencies with a good track record.** A reliable surrogacy agency will have several years' worth of positive feedback from other families. Remember that in some states, commercial surrogacy is illegal. In the UK, paying surrogate mothers is prohibited; you only take care of her expenses during her pregnancy and delivery.

5. **Using websites to find surrogate mothers is also a possible option.** There are online sites where the profiles and photos of potential surrogates may be found. You can apply and choose the nationality and age of your prospect online. Be cautious about getting into binding agreements online, however. Remember to watch out for scam sites. Verify with your lawyer before paying for anything.

6. **Consult with your doctor about your surrogacy options.** Your doctor knows best about your health condition, so he or she can suggest the method that can work best for you.

7. **Legal guidance is important.** You can't successfully conclude the surrogacy process without legal counsel. Legal fees may seem like an unnecessary expense to some, but it's crucial that you have a lawyer to guide you through the intricacies of surrogacy. This will assure that there will be no legal issues during and after the process.

8. **Make use of health insurance to lessen costs.** Purchasing insurance for your surrogate mother can help in reducing the cost of medical bills.

9. **Never rely on an oral agreement even if the surrogate mother is a relative.** Always prepare a carefully written contract duly signed by all parties. Some families are reluctant to ask relatives to sign legal documents, because they don't want to come across as distrusting. Just tell your surrogate that it is for everyone's protection.

10. **Listen to your instinct.** Aside from ensuring that the surrogate mother meets the requirements, you must also listen to your maternal instinct when choosing the surrogate mother-to-be of your child.

11. **You can opt for anonymous donors.** You have the option to use anonymous donors, but be sure that these are from reliable and legitimate ovum and sperm banks.

12. **It helps if surrogate mothers are optimists.** Many people still don't recognize the power of positive thinking in any endeavor. If the surrogate mother has a positive frame of mind, this can affect the baby's condition inside her womb. Research has proven that depressed and unhappy mothers transmit these feelings to the fetus, causing fetal distress.

Conclusion

Wanting to have a baby and a family is a noble endeavor. If you strongly feel that surrogacy is the right option for you, then go for it! However, remember to remain level-headed and refer to the steps and pointers presented in this book to ensure that you are covered and ready should any challenges rise later on.

Your choice of a surrogate mother will impact your baby considerably so choose with prudence, wisely and conscientiously. It's important to note that in traditional surrogacy, the baby inherits the genes of the surrogate mother.

If you and your partner want to be the sole source of the genes inherited by your baby, you can opt for gestational surrogacy. This will allow your baby to inherit both of your genes, and the surrogate mother will only act as the carrier of your baby.

Seek counsel from your lawyer and healthcare professional throughout the decision-making process—and beyond. Let them know how things are progressing on a regular basis, so they can help prevent or address snags before they become full-blown problems.

Your chosen surrogate mother will always be part of your child's history, so give her the care and credit due to her. My best wishes go to your new family!

Finally, I'd like to thank you for purchasing this book! If you found it helpful, I'd greatly appreciate it if you'd take a moment to leave a review on Amazon. Thank you!

78749936R00029

Made in the USA
San Bernardino, CA
08 June 2018